Chapter 1: Understanding Mumps

Overview of Mumps

Mumps is a contagious viral infection caused by the mumps virus, which primarily affects the salivary glands, particularly the parotid glands located near the jaw. The classic symptom of mumps is swollen cheeks and jaw, resulting from inflammation in these glands. While mumps is often associated with childhood, it can affect individuals of any age who are not vaccinated. Understanding mumps is crucial for parents, as it highlights the importance of vaccination and awareness to prevent outbreaks and complications.

Vaccination against mumps is typically achieved through the measles, mumps, and rubella (MMR) vaccine, which is administered in two doses during early childhood. The introduction of the MMR vaccine has significantly reduced the incidence of mumps in many countries; however, outbreaks can still occur, especially in communities with low vaccination rates. Parents play a vital role in safeguarding their children by ensuring they are vaccinated on schedule, thereby contributing to herd immunity and protecting those who cannot be vaccinated due to medical reasons.

Historically, mumps has caused significant morbidity, particularly before the widespread use of the MMR vaccine. Epidemics of mumps have led to severe health complications, including orchitis, oophoritis, and, in rare cases, meningitis or encephalitis. These complications can have long-term effects on health and well-being. Understanding the historical impact of mumps epidemics underscores the need for continued vaccination efforts and awareness to prevent a resurgence of this once-common childhood illness.

In addition to vaccination, strategies for responding to mumps outbreaks include timely identification and isolation of infected individuals, raising awareness in affected communities, and ensuring that those who are at higher risk, such as immunocompromised individuals, receive appropriate preventive measures. Mumps poses a greater risk to these populations, as their immune systems may not effectively combat the virus. Parents should be informed about these risks and the importance of seeking medical advice for their children, especially if they have underlying health conditions.

Finally, misinformation and myths surrounding mumps and vaccination can hinder public health efforts. It is essential for parents to seek reliable information from trusted sources, such as healthcare providers and public health organizations, to dispel myths and understand the benefits of vaccination. Awareness of how mumps can spread, particularly in settings like international travel or crowded environments, is crucial. By staying informed, parents can protect their families and contribute to the broader effort of preventing mumps and its complications in the community.

Symptoms and Diagnosis

Symptoms of mumps typically appear about 14 to 18 days after exposure to the virus. The most recognizable symptom is the swelling of the parotid glands, which are located near the jawline, resulting in the characteristic "chipmunk-like" appearance. This swelling can be accompanied by pain, especially when chewing or swallowing. Other common symptoms include fever, headache, muscle aches, fatigue, and loss of appetite. In some cases, individuals may experience mild respiratory symptoms, such as a runny nose, which can lead to confusion with other viral infections. Parents should remain vigilant and monitor their children for these symptoms, particularly in areas experiencing mumps outbreaks.

Diagnosing mumps can be challenging, especially in the early stages when symptoms may resemble those of other viral infections. Health care providers typically rely on a combination of clinical examination and patient history to assess whether mumps is a possibility. The presence of swollen salivary glands, especially in a previously healthy child, can be a strong indicator. Laboratory tests, such as serology to detect antibodies or polymerase chain reaction

(PCR) tests to identify the virus from saliva or urine, can confirm the diagnosis. It is essential for parents to seek prompt medical attention if they suspect mumps, as timely diagnosis can help prevent further transmission.

In some cases, mumps can lead to complications that may affect the severity of the illness and the overall health of the child. While many individuals recover without issues, complications can include orchitis, which is inflammation of the testicles, and oophoritis, inflammation of the ovaries. Other potential complications include meningitis and encephalitis, both of which can have serious long-term consequences. In immunocompromised populations, the risk of severe disease and complications increases significantly. Parents should be aware of these risks, particularly if their child has underlying health issues or if they are in close contact with individuals who are immunocompromised.

Preventing mumps transmission is crucial, particularly during outbreaks. Vaccination remains the most effective strategy, with the MMR (measles, mumps, rubella) vaccine recommended for children at 12 to 15 months of age, followed by a booster dose between ages 4 and 6. In addition to vaccination, practicing good hygiene, such as frequent handwashing and avoiding close contact with infected individuals, can further reduce the risk of spreading the virus. Parents should also educate their children about the importance of not sharing utensils, drinks, or personal items that could facilitate transmission.

In the context of international travel, awareness of mumps risk becomes even more critical. Outbreaks can occur in various parts of the world, and travelers may be at higher risk, especially if they are not fully vaccinated. Parents planning to travel should consult with their healthcare provider to ensure that their children are up to date on vaccinations and discuss any additional precautions. By understanding the symptoms and diagnosis of mumps, parents can take proactive measures to protect their families and contribute to broader public health efforts aimed at reducing the incidence of this infectious disease.

Historical Impact of Mumps Epidemics

Historical accounts of mumps epidemics reveal significant patterns in public health challenges and responses over the decades. Mumps, caused by the mumps virus, has been a recognized disease for centuries, with documented outbreaks tracing back to the late 19th century. These epidemics often resulted in a high incidence of cases, particularly among children, underscoring the need for effective public health interventions. Communities frequently faced disruptions as schools closed and families isolated sick individuals, highlighting the social and economic impacts of mumps outbreaks.

The introduction of the mumps vaccine in the 1960s marked a transformative moment in the fight against this disease. Prior to vaccination efforts, mumps was a common childhood illness, often leading to complications such as orchitis, meningitis, and, in rare cases, permanent deafness. The widespread implementation of vaccination programs drastically reduced the incidence of mumps, leading to a significant decline in both the number of cases and the severity of complications associated with the disease. This shift demonstrated the power of vaccination in altering the course of infectious diseases and protecting public health.

Despite the advancements brought by vaccination, mumps outbreaks have persisted into the 21st century. In recent years, clusters of mumps cases have emerged in various regions, particularly among populations with lower vaccination rates. These outbreaks serve as a reminder of the importance of maintaining high immunization coverage and addressing vaccine hesitancy. The resurgence of mumps has prompted public health officials to re-evaluate strategies for outbreak response, emphasizing the need for rapid identification of cases, contact tracing, and community education to mitigate the spread of the virus.

The historical impact of mumps epidemics also extends to vulnerable populations, including those who are immunocompromised. Individuals with weakened immune systems may experience more severe manifestations of mumps, making it crucial for surrounding communities to achieve herd immunity through comprehensive vaccination efforts. Public health policies must prioritize these at-risk groups, ensuring that preventive measures are in place. This approach not only protects the vulnerable but also reinforces the collective responsibility of society in combating infectious diseases.

Myths and misinformation surrounding mumps and its vaccination have contributed to public reluctance in some areas, further complicating efforts to achieve high vaccination rates. Historical lessons from past mumps epidemics highlight the need for clear, accurate information about the disease, its transmission, and the benefits of vaccination. By addressing misconceptions and fostering open dialogues about vaccine safety and efficacy, parents can play a pivotal role in promoting awareness and encouraging protective measures within their communities. This proactive stance not only honors the lessons of history but also builds a healthier future for the next generation.

Chapter 2: The Importance of Vaccination

Mumps Vaccination Guidelines

Mumps vaccination guidelines are essential for parents seeking to protect their children from this contagious viral infection. The primary vaccine recommended for mumps prevention is the measles, mumps, and rubella (MMR) vaccine. The Centers for Disease Control and Prevention (CDC) advises that children receive their first dose of the MMR vaccine between 12 and 15 months of age, followed by a second dose between 4 and 6 years. These timing recommendations align with the immune system's development, ensuring that children gain optimal protection against mumps and its associated complications.

Parents should be aware that while mumps vaccination is crucial, it is not a one-time event. The two-dose schedule is designed to provide maximum immunity, as the first dose may not be sufficient for all children. The second dose significantly enhances protection and is particularly important in the context of mumps outbreaks, which can occur even in vaccinated populations. During such outbreaks, health authorities may recommend additional doses or targeted vaccination campaigns to curb transmission effectively.

Mumps can pose serious risks, particularly for certain groups, such as immunocompromised individuals. Parents of children with weakened immune systems should consult healthcare providers to determine the appropriateness of the MMR vaccine. In some cases, alternative vaccination strategies may be necessary to ensure safety while still offering protection against mumps. Furthermore, parents should be informed about the signs and symptoms of mumps, as early diagnosis and treatment can help mitigate complications.

International travel is another critical consideration in mumps vaccination guidelines. Parents planning to travel abroad should check the vaccination status of their children, as some countries may have higher mumps incidence rates. The CDC recommends that children traveling internationally receive the MMR vaccine if they are between 6 and 11 months old, with a follow-up vaccination at the standard age of 12 months. This proactive approach helps safeguard children from potential exposure to mumps during travel, particularly in areas experiencing outbreaks.

Mumps-related myths and misinformation can often lead to vaccine hesitancy. Parents must seek credible information from reliable sources to make informed decisions about vaccinations. Public health campaigns aimed at dispelling myths around the MMR vaccine, including its safety and the actual risks associated with mumps, are crucial in promoting vaccination awareness. By understanding the importance of mumps vaccination and adhering to established guidelines, parents can play a pivotal role in protecting their children and contributing to community health.

Effectiveness of the MMR Vaccine

The effectiveness of the MMR vaccine, which protects against measles, mumps, and rubella, is a critical aspect of public health and individual well-being. Clinical studies have consistently shown that the MMR vaccine provides strong immunity against mumps, significantly reducing the incidence of the disease. Vaccination not only protects the vaccinated individual but also contributes to herd immunity, which is vital for protecting those who cannot be vaccinated, such as infants or individuals with compromised immune systems. Understanding the vaccine's effectiveness can empower parents in making informed decisions regarding their children's health.

After the introduction of the MMR vaccine in the 1970s, the incidence of mumps in vaccinated populations dramatically decreased. Prior to widespread vaccination, mumps was a common childhood illness with a high rate of complications, including orchitis, oophoritis, and, in rare cases, meningitis. The decline in mumps cases following the vaccine's introduction is a testament to its effectiveness. In communities with high vaccination coverage, outbreaks of mumps have become increasingly rare, underscoring the importance of maintaining high immunization rates to prevent resurgence.

Despite its proven effectiveness, some parents remain hesitant about vaccination due to misinformation and myths surrounding the MMR vaccine. Debunking these myths is crucial for increasing vaccine uptake. Research has shown that the MMR vaccine does not cause autism, a claim that has been thoroughly discredited. By educating themselves and others about the safety and benefits of the vaccine, parents can help combat the false narratives that threaten public health and contribute to vaccine hesitancy.

The effectiveness of the MMR vaccine is also evident in outbreak response strategies. When mumps cases do occur, vaccination remains a key tool in controlling the spread of the virus. Public health officials often emphasize the importance of vaccination during outbreaks, encouraging individuals who are unvaccinated or under-vaccinated to receive their doses. This proactive approach not only helps to contain outbreaks but also reassures parents about the importance of keeping their children up to date on vaccinations to protect their community.

Finally, understanding the long-term impact of mumps and its complications reinforces the necessity of the MMR vaccine. Mumps can lead to serious health issues, particularly in immunocompromised populations. Vaccination reduces the risk of these complications and helps safeguard the health of vulnerable individuals. By recognizing the broader implications of mumps and the vital role of the MMR vaccine in prevention, parents can make informed choices that contribute to their children's health and the well-being of their communities.

Addressing Vaccination Hesitancy

Addressing vaccination hesitancy is a crucial part of ensuring that children are protected against mumps and other preventable diseases.

Many parents may have concerns or doubts about the necessity and safety of vaccines, often fueled by misinformation. It is essential for parents to understand the scientific evidence supporting vaccinations, particularly in the context of mumps, a disease that can lead to serious complications such as meningitis and orchitis. By providing accurate information and addressing common misconceptions, parents can make informed decisions that contribute to their children's health and the well-being of the community.

One significant factor contributing to vaccination hesitancy is the prevalence of myths surrounding vaccines. Misconceptions about the risks associated with vaccinations may stem from anecdotal reports or misinformation spread through social media. For instance, some parents may believe that the MMR (measles, mumps, rubella) vaccine leads to developmental disorders, a claim that has been thoroughly debunked by scientific research. By openly discussing these myths and providing evidence-based responses, parents can better understand the importance of vaccination as a critical tool in preventing outbreaks and protecting vulnerable populations.

The historical impact of mumps epidemics highlights the necessity of vaccination. Before the widespread use of the MMR vaccine, mumps was a common childhood illness that could lead to severe complications. Outbreaks not only affected individual health but also strained healthcare systems and caused significant societal disruption. Understanding the consequences of past epidemics can serve as a powerful reminder of the importance of maintaining high vaccination rates to prevent a resurgence of mumps. By learning from history, parents can appreciate the role that vaccines play in safeguarding public health.

Additionally, addressing the unique challenges faced by immunocompromised populations is vital in discussions about vaccination. Children with weakened immune systems may be at greater risk for severe mumps complications. Educating parents about the importance of vaccinating healthy children helps create herd immunity, which protects those who cannot be vaccinated due to medical conditions. By emphasizing the collective responsibility of vaccination, parents can be encouraged to see their decision not just as a personal choice but as a contribution to community health.

In conclusion, fostering a supportive environment where parents can discuss their concerns about vaccination is essential. Providing clear, factual information about mumps, the benefits of vaccination, and the potential risks of not vaccinating can help alleviate fears. Encouraging dialogue between parents, healthcare providers, and public health officials can build trust and create a more informed community, ultimately leading to higher vaccination rates and better protection against mumps and its associated complications.

Chapter 3: Mumps Outbreak Response Strategies

Recognizing an Outbreak

Recognizing an outbreak of mumps is crucial for parents to ensure the health and safety of their children and community. Mumps is a highly contagious viral infection that primarily affects children but can also impact adolescents and adults. The signs of an outbreak often begin with a series of confirmed cases within a close-knit community, such as schools or daycare centers. Parents should be vigilant for symptoms such as fever, swelling of the salivary glands, headache, and muscle aches. The presence of these symptoms, especially in conjunction with reported cases in the area, can indicate an outbreak is occurring.

Monitoring local health department announcements and being aware of the vaccination status of your child is essential. Health officials typically release information about confirmed cases, vaccination rates, and recommendations for parents. An outbreak is often declared when there are multiple confirmed cases in a specific geographic area, especially if there are unvaccinated individuals involved. Awareness of these developments helps parents take proactive measures to protect their children, such as reinforcing vaccination schedules or minimizing exposure to potential carriers.

In addition to recognizing immediate symptoms, parents should be informed about the historical context of mumps outbreaks. Past epidemics have highlighted the vulnerabilities of populations with lower vaccination rates. Understanding how mumps spread and the conditions that facilitate outbreaks can empower parents to engage in community health efforts. For instance, during previous outbreaks, communities with higher vaccination rates experienced milder effects, emphasizing the importance of herd immunity. Parents are pivotal in advocating for vaccination and educating others about the benefits of immunization against mumps.

Parents of immunocompromised children should be particularly aware of mumps outbreaks. These children are at a higher risk for complications, such as meningitis and orchitis, which can lead to long-term health issues. During an outbreak, parents must take extra precautions, including discussing their child's health needs with a healthcare provider and considering additional protective measures. It is vital to communicate with schools and community organizations to ensure that appropriate strategies are in place to protect vulnerable populations.

Lastly, dispelling myths and misinformation surrounding mumps and its vaccination is critical for outbreak recognition and response. Many misconceptions about mumps and the vaccine can lead to hesitancy and lower vaccination rates, making communities more susceptible to outbreaks. Parents should seek information from reputable sources and engage in discussions with healthcare professionals to better understand the risks associated with mumps and the benefits of vaccination. By fostering informed conversations and sharing accurate information, parents can play a significant role in reducing the incidence of mumps and enhancing public health efforts in their communities.

Community Preparedness

Community preparedness is a crucial aspect of managing mumps outbreaks, especially considering the potential for rapid transmission in close-knit environments like schools and daycare centers. Parents play a vital role in this process, as they are often the first line of defense when it comes to recognizing symptoms and understanding the importance of vaccination. By fostering awareness within their communities, parents can help ensure that others are informed about mumps and the preventive measures that can be taken. This collective effort can significantly reduce the likelihood of outbreaks, protecting not only individual families but the broader community as well.

To effectively prepare for a possible mumps outbreak, parents should educate themselves and their networks about the signs and symptoms of mumps, which include fever, headache, and swelling of the salivary glands. Recognizing these symptoms early can lead to prompt diagnosis and treatment, thereby minimizing the risk of spreading the virus. Additionally, parents should advocate for vaccination, as the MMR (measles, mumps, rubella) vaccine is the most effective way to prevent mumps. By ensuring that their children are vaccinated on schedule, parents contribute to herd immunity, protecting those who are unable to be vaccinated due to medical conditions.

In the event of an outbreak, a coordinated response is essential. Parents should be familiar with local public health policies and guidelines regarding mumps. This knowledge allows them to understand the measures that may be implemented, such as temporary school closures or quarantine protocols. Communication with local health departments can provide valuable information on the outbreak's status and recommended actions. Parents should also be prepared to share this information with other caregivers and family members to ensure everyone is informed and compliant with health advisories.

Community preparedness also involves addressing the misinformation surrounding mumps and vaccines. Many myths and misconceptions can lead to vaccine hesitancy, which poses a significant risk during outbreaks. Parents can take the initiative to debunk these myths by sharing accurate information from reputable sources, such as the Centers for Disease Control and Prevention (CDC) and the World Health Organization (WHO). Engaging in conversations about the safety and effectiveness of vaccines can help alleviate fears and encourage others to protect themselves and their children.

Finally, parents should consider the implications of mumps outbreaks on international travel. With increased global connectivity, the risk of mumps spreading across borders is heightened. Before traveling, parents should ensure their children are fully vaccinated and inquire about the vaccination requirements of their destination. Understanding the local prevalence of mumps and associated health risks in other countries can help families make informed decisions about their travel plans, further contributing to community preparedness on a global scale.

Role of Schools and Institutions

Schools and institutions play a pivotal role in shaping the health and well-being of children, particularly regarding the prevention and management of diseases like mumps. As centers of learning and social interaction, schools are essential in promoting vaccination awareness and ensuring that children are protected against infectious diseases. By fostering an environment that prioritizes health education, schools can help dispel myths and misinformation about mumps and other vaccine-preventable diseases. This not only informs parents about the importance of vaccinations but also encourages children to understand their role in preventing the spread of infections.

In the event of a mumps outbreak, schools are often on the front line of response strategies. They serve as critical points for communication between health authorities, parents, and the community. Schools must have clear protocols in place to manage outbreaks effectively, including timely notification of parents about potential exposure and guidelines for vaccination status. By collaborating with local health departments, schools can implement strategies to contain outbreaks, such as temporary closures or increased health screenings, ensuring that the health of students and staff is prioritized.

The historical impact of mumps epidemics underscores the importance of vigilant health policies within educational institutions. Past outbreaks have demonstrated how quickly mumps can spread in crowded environments, highlighting the need for effective monitoring and vaccination programs. Schools can take proactive measures by requiring proof of vaccination for enrollment, thus creating a safer environment for all students. Furthermore, educational institutions can serve as platforms for historical education, helping children and parents understand the consequences of past epidemics and the importance of vaccination in preventing similar occurrences.

Mumps can have severe complications, particularly in immunocompromised populations, making awareness and education in schools crucial. Children with weakened immune systems may be at a higher risk for serious health issues resulting from mumps infection. Schools must work to ensure that all students, especially those at higher risk, are protected through vaccination and that they have access to necessary resources and support. By fostering a culture of inclusivity and health awareness, schools can help mitigate the risks associated with mumps for vulnerable populations.

In an increasingly interconnected world, the implications of mumps extend beyond local communities, particularly concerning international travel. Schools that educate families about the risks of mumps during travel can empower parents to make informed decisions regarding vaccinations before embarking on trips. By providing resources and information about mumps transmission prevention methods, schools can help equip parents and students with the knowledge they need to protect themselves, both locally and abroad. Through comprehensive health education programs, schools can play a vital role in ensuring the well-being of students and the broader community in the face of ongoing public health challenges related to mumps.

Chapter 4: Mumps Complications and Long-Term Effects

Common Complications of Mumps

Mumps is a viral illness that can lead to several complications, some of which may have lasting effects on an individual's health. While many people associate mumps with its characteristic swollen salivary glands, the virus can affect other parts of the body and result in more serious health issues. Parents should be aware of these potential complications to understand the importance of vaccination and prompt medical attention if symptoms arise.

One of the most common complications of mumps is orchitis, which is inflammation of the testicles. This condition occurs in approximately one-third of post-pubertal males who contract mumps. Orchitis can lead to significant pain and swelling, and in some cases, it may result in reduced fertility or even infertility. Parents of boys should be particularly vigilant about mumps symptoms and the importance of vaccination, as the consequences of orchitis can have long-term implications.

Another serious complication is encephalitis, an inflammation of the brain that can occur in rare cases following a mumps infection. Symptoms of encephalitis may include headache, fever, confusion, and seizures. While the risk of developing encephalitis from mumps is low, the condition can lead to neurological damage, learning disabilities, or other cognitive impairments. Understanding the potential for such complications underscores the need for preventative measures, including vaccination, especially in areas experiencing outbreaks.

Mumps can also lead to complications such as meningitis, which is the inflammation of the protective membranes covering the brain and spinal cord. Mumps meningitis can result in severe headaches, fever, and neck stiffness. Although many individuals recover completely, there is a risk of long-term effects, including hearing loss and cognitive challenges. Awareness of these risks can help parents make informed decisions regarding vaccination and the importance of seeking medical care if their child exhibits symptoms of mumps.

In immunocompromised populations, the risks associated with mumps complications are heightened. Individuals with weakened immune systems may experience more severe symptoms and complications from mumps, highlighting the importance of vaccination in protecting these vulnerable groups. Parents should be aware of the heightened risks for their children or family members who may be immunocompromised and engage in discussions with healthcare providers to develop appropriate prevention strategies. Understanding the potential complications of mumps can empower parents to advocate for vaccination and proactive health measures within their communities.

Long-Term Health Consequences

Long-term health consequences of mumps can be significant, affecting not only the individual who contracts the virus but also their family and community. Mumps is primarily known for its immediate symptoms, such as fever and swollen salivary glands, but the potential for long-term complications is a critical aspect that every parent should understand. While mumps is often perceived as a mild childhood illness, it can lead to severe health issues, particularly in vulnerable populations. Awareness of these consequences is essential for informed decision-making regarding vaccination and prevention strategies.

One of the most concerning complications of mumps is viral meningitis, which can occur when the virus spreads to the central nervous system. This condition can lead to long-term neurological effects, including cognitive impairments and seizures. Although the risk of developing viral meningitis from mumps is relatively low, the potential for serious outcomes makes it imperative for parents to recognize the importance of vaccination. Additionally, mumps can lead to orchitis in post-pubertal males, resulting in complications such as infertility. Understanding these risks can motivate parents to advocate for timely vaccinations for their children.

Hearing loss is another significant long-term consequence associated with mumps infection. Although it is a rare complication, it can occur in both children and adults who contract the virus. Mumps-related hearing loss may be unilateral or bilateral, and the severity can vary. This complication can have profound effects on a child's development, education, and social interactions. Parents should be aware that the risk of hearing loss, although not common, underscores the importance of preventive measures, including vaccination, to protect their children from mumps and its potential aftermath.

Immunocompromised individuals are particularly at risk for severe mumps complications. For children with weakened immune systems, such as those undergoing cancer treatment or living with chronic conditions, mumps can pose a serious threat. These children may experience more severe symptoms and a higher likelihood of long-term health issues, making vaccination even more crucial for their protection. Parents of immunocompromised children should be proactive in discussing vaccination options and outbreak responses with their healthcare providers to ensure their children are safeguarded against the virus.

Finally, understanding the historical impact of mumps epidemics can also inform parents about the long-term health consequences. Past outbreaks have highlighted not only the immediate health threats posed by the virus but also the strain on public health systems, and the lasting effects on individuals who suffered complications. Public health policies have evolved to prioritize mumps vaccination, reflecting the importance of prevention in averting these long-term consequences. By understanding the historical context and potential complications associated with mumps, parents can make better-informed decisions about vaccination and advocate for the health of their children and communities.

Special Considerations for Vulnerable Populations

Special considerations for vulnerable populations are crucial in understanding and addressing the impact of mumps outbreaks. Vulnerable groups, including infants, the elderly, and individuals with weakened immune systems, require specific attention to ensure their safety and well-being. Parents must be aware of the unique risks these populations face when it comes to mumps transmission and complications, as well as the importance of vaccination in preventing outbreaks.

Infants under one year of age are particularly susceptible to mumps, as they may not yet have received their first dose of the measles, mumps, and rubella (MMR) vaccine, which is typically administered between 12 and 15 months of age. In addition to being unvaccinated, infants also have underdeveloped immune systems, making them more vulnerable to severe mumps complications, such as meningitis and orchitis. Parents should consider the risks associated with exposure to mumps in environments where outbreaks are occurring and discuss the possibility of earlier vaccination with their healthcare providers if they anticipate travel or exposure to outbreaks.

Elderly individuals, especially those who have not been vaccinated or have received their vaccinations many years ago, may also face significant risks. While mumps is often viewed as a childhood illness, adults can contract it and experience more severe symptoms and complications. Parents should be aware of the importance of ensuring that older family members are protected through vaccination and boosted if necessary. This awareness is especially pertinent in family gatherings or community settings where mumps may be circulating.

Immunocompromised populations, including those undergoing cancer treatment, organ transplant recipients, and individuals with autoimmune disorders, are at heightened risk for severe mumps infections. The immune system's ability to respond to the virus is compromised, potentially leading to more severe disease and complications. Parents must advocate for vaccination among their children, while also ensuring that their own health practices minimize the risk of transmission to vulnerable family members, such as avoiding exposure in crowded places during outbreaks.

Finally, public health policy plays a significant role in protecting vulnerable populations from mumps outbreaks. Parents should stay informed about local vaccination rates and outbreak reports in their communities. Engaging with public health initiatives and understanding the importance of herd immunity can help protect those who cannot be vaccinated, such as infants and immunocompromised individuals. By fostering a culture of awareness and proactive health measures, parents can contribute to the reduction of mumps transmission and safeguard the health of their families and communities.

Chapter 5: Mumps in Immunocompromised Populations

Understanding Immunocompromised States

Immunocompromised states refer to conditions that weaken the immune system, making individuals more susceptible to infections, including mumps. For parents, understanding these states is crucial, especially when considering vaccination and prevention strategies for their children. Various factors can lead to an immunocompromised state, such as congenital immunodeficiencies, chronic illnesses like diabetes or cancer, and medical treatments such as chemotherapy or immunosuppressive drugs. These conditions can significantly affect how the body responds to vaccines, including the MMR (measles, mumps, rubella) vaccine, and may necessitate special considerations for the health and safety of affected children.

Children with weakened immune systems are at a higher risk for contracting mumps and experiencing more severe complications. Mumps, while often seen as a mild childhood illness, can lead to serious health issues such as meningitis, orchitis, and hearing loss, particularly in those with compromised immunity. Parents should be particularly vigilant if their child is immunocompromised, as the typical vaccine schedule may not apply. Consulting healthcare providers for personalized advice regarding vaccination and prevention methods is essential for minimizing risks and ensuring the best health outcomes.

Preventing mumps transmission in immunocompromised populations is vital, especially during outbreaks. Parents should be informed about the importance of herd immunity; when a significant portion of the population is vaccinated, it helps protect those who cannot be vaccinated or who may not respond adequately to vaccines. Strategies to prevent mumps transmission include frequent handwashing, avoiding close contact with infected individuals, and maintaining up-to-date vaccinations for healthy family members. In situations where outbreaks occur, schools and communities may implement additional measures, such as temporary exclusion from school or daycare for unvaccinated or immunocompromised children.

International travel can also pose unique challenges for immunocompromised children regarding mumps exposure. Different countries have varying vaccination rates and outbreaks of vaccine-preventable diseases, including mumps. Parents planning travel should consult with healthcare providers to assess the risk of exposure, discuss the necessity of additional vaccinations, and implement health precautions, such as avoiding crowded places and practicing good hygiene. Being aware of the health status of the destination country can help parents make informed decisions to protect their children.

Mumps vaccination awareness is a key component in safeguarding not only immunocompromised children but the broader community. Parents should be equipped with accurate information about the MMR vaccine, including its efficacy, safety, and the importance of maintaining high vaccination rates to prevent outbreaks. Combating myths and misinformation surrounding vaccines is crucial, as misconceptions can lead to hesitancy and decreased vaccination coverage. By advocating for informed decisions and sharing knowledge about the implications of mumps in immunocompromised individuals, parents can play a pivotal role in protecting their children and contributing to public health efforts.

Risks Associated with Mumps

Mumps is a viral infection that can lead to a range of complications, posing significant risks, particularly for children and certain vulnerable populations. While many may associate mumps with mild symptoms like swollen salivary glands, the reality is that the virus can cause serious health issues. Parents should be aware that mumps can lead to complications such as orchitis, which is inflammation of the testicles, and oophoritis, inflammation of the ovaries. These complications can result in long-term reproductive health concerns, making early awareness and prevention essential.

Another critical risk associated with mumps is the potential for meningitis, an infection of the protective membranes covering the brain and spinal cord. This condition can lead to severe neurological complications, including seizures and cognitive impairments. In some cases, mumps can also result in encephalitis, a more severe brain inflammation that can have lasting effects. Understanding these risks highlights the importance of vaccination, which significantly reduces the likelihood of contracting mumps and its associated complications.

Immunocompromised individuals face heightened risks if they contract mumps. This includes children undergoing cancer treatment, those with autoimmune disorders, and individuals who have received organ transplants. The immune system's compromised state makes it more difficult to fight off infections, leading to a higher incidence of severe complications. Parents with immunocompromised children should be particularly vigilant about vaccination and herd immunity, as outbreaks can pose serious threats to their health.

Furthermore, mumps can have implications for public health, particularly during outbreaks. The spread of mumps in schools and community settings highlights the importance of vaccination and effective outbreak response strategies. Public health policies play a crucial role in managing mumps outbreaks, including vaccination campaigns and educational initiatives to counter misinformation. Parents must remain informed and proactive in advocating for vaccination within their communities to protect their children and reduce the risk of outbreaks.

Lastly, myths and misinformation surrounding mumps and its vaccination can lead to hesitancy and increased risk of infection. It is essential for parents to seek reliable information and understand the benefits of vaccination not only for their children but also for the community as a whole. Addressing these myths through education can help promote a culture of vaccination, safeguarding everyone, especially those at higher risk from mumps complications. Awareness of these risks and the importance of vaccination is crucial for ensuring the health and safety of children and the broader community.

Preventive Measures for At-Risk Individuals

Preventive measures play a crucial role in safeguarding at-risk individuals from mumps, particularly as awareness around this disease becomes increasingly vital for parents. At-risk individuals include those who are unvaccinated, have underlying health conditions, or are immunocompromised. Ensuring that these groups are adequately protected requires a multifaceted approach that combines vaccination, education, and vigilant monitoring of health conditions. Parents must prioritize vaccinations for their children and ensure that they are up to date on the recommended immunization schedule, which includes the measles, mumps, and rubella (MMR) vaccine. This vaccine is highly effective in preventing mumps and is critical for creating herd immunity within communities.

In addition to vaccination, parents should be educated about the importance of recognizing the early signs and symptoms of mumps. Symptoms such as fever, muscle aches, and notably swollen salivary glands can appear within two to three weeks after exposure. Early detection can significantly reduce the risk of complications and transmission to others. Parents should maintain open communication with their children about hygiene practices, such as frequent handwashing and avoiding sharing personal items, which can help mitigate the spread of mumps, especially in communal settings like schools and daycare centers.

For families with immunocompromised members, extra precautions are necessary. This may involve limiting exposure to potential outbreaks and closely monitoring public health advisories regarding mumps outbreaks in the community. Parents should consult healthcare providers to discuss tailored vaccination strategies, as some individuals may not be eligible for the standard MMR vaccine due to their health conditions. These discussions can provide insight into alternative protective measures that can be implemented to ensure the safety of vulnerable family members.

When it comes to international travel, parents should be particularly vigilant. Mumps is still prevalent in various parts of the world, and travelers can unknowingly bring the virus back to their home countries. Prior to traveling, parents should consult with a healthcare professional to ensure that their children are vaccinated according to the destination's health guidelines. It is also advisable to familiarize oneself with potential health risks in the destination country and consider additional preventive measures, such as avoiding crowded places and practicing good hygiene during travel.

Finally, addressing myths and misinformation about mumps and its vaccination is essential for effective prevention. Parents should seek reliable sources of information and engage in discussions with healthcare professionals to debunk common misconceptions about the MMR vaccine and its safety. Educating oneself and others can foster a community that prioritizes public health and encourages vaccination, ultimately protecting at-risk individuals from the complications of mumps. By taking proactive steps, parents can help create a safe environment for their children and the broader community, reducing the likelihood of outbreaks and ensuring that the historical impact of mumps epidemics is not repeated.

Chapter 6: Preventing Mumps Transmission

Hygiene Practices

Hygiene practices play a critical role in preventing the transmission of mumps, an illness that can lead to serious complications, particularly in unvaccinated populations. Parents should understand the importance of maintaining good hygiene not only to protect their children but also to contribute to the broader community's health. Simple measures such as regular handwashing can significantly reduce the risk of spreading the virus. Encourage your children to wash their hands thoroughly with soap and water, especially after coughing, sneezing, or playing outside, as these are common times when germs can be transferred.

In addition to handwashing, teaching children to avoid close contact with individuals who exhibit symptoms of mumps is essential. This includes maintaining a safe distance from those who are ill and refraining from sharing personal items such as utensils, drinks, or towels. Parents should model these behaviors themselves, as children often learn by example. By fostering an environment where hygiene is prioritized, families can help mitigate the risk of mumps outbreaks in their communities.

Understanding the modes of transmission for mumps is crucial for implementing effective hygiene practices. The virus spreads through respiratory droplets when an infected person coughs or sneezes. Therefore, covering one's mouth and nose with a tissue or elbow while sneezing or coughing is a vital practice. Additionally, parents should emphasize the importance of staying home when sick, to prevent spreading the virus to others. This not only protects classmates and family members but also supports public health efforts to control potential outbreaks.

In the context of international travel, hygiene practices become even more significant. Parents planning trips should ensure their children are up to date on vaccinations, including the mumps vaccine, before traveling to areas where outbreaks may be occurring. Alongside vaccination, travelers should prioritize hygiene by frequently washing hands, using hand sanitizer, and avoiding crowded places, especially in regions known for mumps cases. These precautions can help safeguard not only their children but also other travelers and locals.

Finally, addressing mumps-related myths and misinformation is crucial for promoting effective hygiene practices. Some may believe that mumps is no longer a significant concern due to widespread vaccination efforts. However, outbreaks can still occur, particularly in under-vaccinated communities. Educating families about the continuing relevance of hygiene and vaccination in preventing mumps is vital. By fostering a culture of awareness and proactive hygiene practices, parents can help protect their children and contribute to the overall health of their communities.

Isolation During Outbreaks

During outbreaks of mumps, isolation becomes a crucial strategy to control the spread of the virus, particularly among unvaccinated individuals or those who have weakened immune systems. Parents should understand the importance of isolation not only for the health of their children but also for the broader community. Mumps is contagious and can spread rapidly through respiratory droplets, making it essential to limit contact with infected individuals. When a case of mumps is confirmed, public health authorities often recommend that infected individuals stay at home and avoid close contact with others, especially those who are unvaccinated or have compromised immune systems.

Implementing isolation measures effectively requires clear communication within families and communities. Parents should be vigilant in monitoring their children for symptoms of mumps, which include fever, swollen salivary glands, and headache. If a child exhibits these signs, prompt medical consultation is vital for diagnosis and to initiate isolation. Parents should educate their children about the importance of staying away from school and social gatherings during an outbreak. This not only reduces the risk of transmission but also reinforces the concept of community responsibility in public health.

Isolation protocols can vary depending on the severity of the outbreak and local health guidelines. Generally, individuals diagnosed with mumps should remain isolated for at least five days after the onset of symptoms. During this period, parents can help manage their child's discomfort with appropriate home care measures, such as ensuring adequate hydration and rest. Additionally, monitoring for any complications, such as orchitis or meningitis, is essential. Open discussions with healthcare providers can help parents navigate these challenges and ensure their child receives the necessary support.

Parents must also consider the impact of isolation on their children's emotional and social well-being. Prolonged isolation can lead to feelings of loneliness and anxiety, especially for school-aged children who may miss out on important social interactions. To mitigate these effects, parents can facilitate virtual playdates or engage in fun home activities that keep their children connected with friends and family while adhering to isolation guidelines. This approach not only distracts from the isolation but also fosters resilience and adaptability in children.

Lastly, parents should be aware of the role that vaccination plays in preventing mumps outbreaks and the need for community-wide immunity. Promoting vaccination among peers is essential to reduce the risk of future outbreaks and the need for isolation. By understanding the significance of isolation during outbreaks, parents can better protect their families and contribute to the overall health of their communities. Continued education about mumps, vaccination awareness, and the importance of public health policies is vital to ensure that families are prepared to respond effectively to mumps and other infectious diseases.

Role of Vaccination in Prevention

Vaccination plays a crucial role in the prevention of mumps, a contagious viral infection that can lead to serious complications, including orchitis, meningitis, and deafness. The introduction of the measles, mumps, and rubella (MMR) vaccine in the 1970s has significantly reduced the incidence of mumps worldwide. By immunizing children at a young age, parents can protect not only their own children but also contribute to herd immunity, which helps shield those who are unable to be vaccinated due to medical reasons. This collective immunity is vital in preventing outbreaks, particularly in communities where vaccine uptake may be lower.

Mumps vaccination is particularly important in the context of recent outbreaks that have occurred in various regions. These outbreaks often stem from clusters of unvaccinated individuals. Public health officials emphasize the need for high vaccination coverage to prevent the spread of mumps, especially in settings such as schools, where children are in close contact. Parents are encouraged to stay informed about vaccination schedules and ensure their children receive both doses of the MMR vaccine, which are most effective when administered on time.

Historically, mumps was responsible for significant morbidity before the advent of the vaccine. Epidemics occurred with regularity, resulting in thousands of hospitalizations each year. The decline in mumps cases due to widespread vaccination has not only reduced the burden of the disease but has also allowed for a better understanding of its complications. Parents should be aware that while mumps is often mild in children, it can have serious long-term effects, particularly in adolescents and adults, making vaccination even more critical.

For certain populations, such as those who are immunocompromised, the risks associated with mumps are heightened. Vaccination is essential for protecting these vulnerable individuals, as they are at greater risk for severe illness and complications. It is important for parents of immunocompromised children to discuss vaccination strategies with their healthcare providers, ensuring that the family takes appropriate precautions to minimize the risk of exposure to mumps and other vaccine-preventable diseases.

In an increasingly interconnected world, international travel poses unique challenges for mumps prevention. Parents planning to travel should be aware of the vaccination requirements and the prevalence of mumps in their destination countries. By ensuring that their children are fully vaccinated before traveling, parents can help prevent the international spread of mumps. Additionally, understanding the myths and misinformation surrounding vaccinations can empower parents to make informed decisions, ultimately contributing to the success of public health policies aimed at eradicating mumps and safeguarding community health.

Chapter 7: Mumps and International Travel

Mumps Risk in Different Regions

Mumps risk varies significantly across different regions, influenced by factors such as vaccination rates, population density, and public health policies. In areas with high vaccination coverage, mumps cases are relatively rare, and outbreaks are infrequent. Conversely, regions with lower vaccination rates often experience higher incidence of mumps, which can lead to significant outbreaks. Parents must understand these regional differences, as they can directly affect their children's health and the overall safety of their communities.

In the United States, for instance, mumps has seen a resurgence in certain communities, particularly where vaccine hesitancy is prevalent. The MMR (measles, mumps, rubella) vaccine is highly effective, yet pockets of unvaccinated individuals can contribute to the spread of the virus. Parents living in these areas should be vigilant and ensure their children are fully vaccinated to reduce the risk of contracting mumps. Awareness of local health trends can help parents make informed decisions regarding vaccinations and other preventive measures.

International travel introduces another layer of risk, as mumps incidence varies globally. Some countries experience endemic mumps, and travelers may inadvertently bring the virus back home. Parents planning international trips should consult travel health advisories and ensure their children are up to date on vaccinations before departure. This is especially crucial for trips to regions where mumps outbreaks are reported, as exposure can lead to infection and subsequent complications.

Public health policies also play a vital role in determining mumps risk in different regions. Countries with strong immunization programs often report lower incidence rates. Conversely, regions with lax vaccination policies or inadequate healthcare infrastructure may face higher risks of outbreaks. Parents should advocate for robust public health initiatives and support policies that promote vaccination to protect not just their own children, but also the wider community.

Lastly, addressing mumps-related myths and misinformation is essential to reducing risk. Misconceptions about vaccine safety and efficacy can deter parents from vaccinating their children, leading to increased vulnerability to mumps. Educational efforts aimed at dispelling these myths are crucial in fostering a better understanding of the importance of vaccination. By arming themselves with accurate information, parents can contribute to a healthier environment for their children and help prevent the spread of mumps in their communities.

Vaccination Requirements for Travel

Vaccination requirements for travel have become increasingly important in the context of public health, particularly concerning diseases like mumps. Many countries have established specific vaccination criteria for travelers, aimed at controlling the spread of infectious diseases. For parents, understanding these requirements is essential not only to ensure compliance with regulations but also to protect their children from potential outbreaks while traveling. Mumps, a contagious viral infection, can have serious complications, making vaccination a critical preventive measure.

Before traveling, parents should be aware of the vaccination policies of their destination. Some countries may require proof of vaccination against mumps, especially if there is an ongoing outbreak or if the traveler is visiting areas with low vaccination rates. This requirement is often part of broader public health strategies designed to maintain herd immunity and protect vulnerable populations. Parents should consult their healthcare providers or the Centers for Disease Control and Prevention (CDC) for the latest travel vaccination recommendations and requirements.

In addition to understanding the requirements, parents must also ensure that their children are up to date on their mumps vaccinations. The MMR vaccine, which protects against measles, mumps, and rubella, is typically administered in two doses during childhood. It is crucial for parents to check their child's vaccination history before embarking on international trips. Having this documentation readily available can help streamline the travel process and provide peace of mind in case of unexpected health checks at borders or during travel.

Traveling with children who are immunocompromised poses additional challenges regarding mumps vaccination. These children may not respond adequately to the vaccine or may be at higher risk of severe complications if they contract the virus. Parents should work closely with healthcare providers to assess the risks and determine the best prevention strategies. In some cases, avoiding non-essential travel to areas with known mumps outbreaks might be the safest course of action.

Lastly, awareness of mumps transmission prevention methods is vital for all travelers, regardless of vaccination status. Parents should educate their children about the importance of good hygiene practices, such as frequent handwashing and avoiding close contact with individuals who exhibit symptoms of mumps. By taking these precautions, families can help minimize the risk of exposure to mumps and other infectious diseases during their travels, ensuring that their adventures are both enjoyable and safe.

Precautions for Traveling Families

Traveling with children can be an enriching experience, but it also requires careful planning, especially in the context of vaccine-preventable diseases like mumps. Families should prioritize mumps vaccination before embarking on any trip, particularly if they are traveling to areas where the disease is more prevalent. Ensuring that all family members, especially children over the age of one, are up to date on their MMR (measles, mumps, rubella) vaccinations will significantly reduce the risk of contracting mumps during travel. Parents should consult with their healthcare provider to review vaccination records and consider any necessary boosters.

Mumps is highly contagious and can spread easily in close quarters, making it essential for families to understand transmission prevention methods while traveling. When in crowded places, such as airports, hotels, or public transport, practicing good hygiene is crucial. Frequent handwashing with soap and water, or using hand sanitizer when soap is unavailable, can help reduce the risk of exposure. Additionally, parents should teach their children about the importance of not sharing personal items and avoiding close contact with individuals who appear ill, as these are common ways mumps can be transmitted.

In the event of a mumps outbreak at a travel destination, families should be prepared to respond quickly. It is advisable for parents to stay informed about any ongoing outbreaks in the areas they plan to visit. This can be done through local health department updates or the Centers for Disease Control and Prevention (CDC) advisories. If an outbreak is reported, families may want to reconsider their travel plans or take extra precautions, such as avoiding crowded events and ensuring access to medical care should symptoms arise. Understanding the symptoms of mumps, which include fever, headache, muscle aches, fatigue, and swollen salivary glands, can aid in early detection and prompt treatment.

For families traveling internationally, the risk of encountering mumps may be heightened, especially in regions with low vaccination coverage. Parents should research the vaccination rates of their travel destinations and consider additional vaccinations for their children if they are traveling to high-risk areas. It is also critical to have a plan in place for accessing healthcare should a family member develop symptoms while abroad. This includes knowing the location of nearby hospitals and clinics, as well as having a basic understanding of the healthcare system in the destination country.

Lastly, addressing mumps-related myths and misinformation is vital for traveling families. Many misconceptions about the safety and necessity of vaccinations can lead to hesitancy in keeping children immunized. Parents should seek reliable information from healthcare professionals and trusted public health sources to ensure they make informed decisions about vaccinations. By being educated and prepared, families can mitigate the risks associated with mumps during travel and enjoy their adventures with greater peace of mind, knowing they have taken the necessary precautions to protect their loved ones.

Chapter 8: Advances in Diagnosis and Treatment

Diagnostic Techniques for Mumps

Diagnostic techniques for mumps play a crucial role in identifying and managing this viral infection, especially in the context of outbreaks and vaccination awareness. The primary method for diagnosing mumps is through clinical evaluation, where healthcare professionals assess the patient's symptoms, such as fever, headache, muscle aches, fatigue, and the characteristic swelling of the parotid glands. Parents should be vigilant in recognizing these symptoms, as early detection can help prevent the spread of the virus among unvaccinated populations and those who may be more vulnerable to complications.

In addition to clinical evaluation, laboratory tests are essential for confirming a mumps diagnosis. The most common test is the detection of mumps virus RNA through reverse transcription polymerase chain reaction (RT-PCR). This test is highly sensitive and can be performed on various samples, including throat swabs and urine. Serological testing, which measures the presence of mumps-specific antibodies in the blood, is also useful, particularly in cases where symptoms have resolved. Understanding these diagnostic techniques empowers parents to seek appropriate medical attention for their children if mumps is suspected.

Rapid and accurate diagnosis of mumps is critical for effective outbreak response strategies. Public health authorities rely on timely data to implement containment measures, such as isolation of infected individuals and vaccination campaigns in affected communities. Parents should be aware that during an outbreak, diagnostic confirmation may be required for their children to return to school or participate in community activities. Being informed about these protocols can help parents navigate the challenges posed by outbreaks and advocate for their children's health.

Moreover, advancements in diagnostic techniques have significantly improved the management of mumps. For instance, the development of rapid diagnostic tests has made it possible to obtain results more quickly, facilitating prompt public health response actions. These advancements not only assist in controlling outbreaks but also enhance the understanding of mumps epidemiology, particularly in immunocompromised populations who may experience atypical presentations or more severe disease. Awareness of these advancements can help parents appreciate the importance of ongoing research in the field of infectious diseases.

As misinformation about mumps and its vaccination continues to circulate, understanding the diagnostic process is vital for parents. Knowledge of how mumps is diagnosed allows parents to critically evaluate the information they encounter and make informed decisions regarding vaccination and healthcare. By staying informed about diagnostic techniques and their implications for public health policy, parents can contribute to community efforts in preventing mumps transmission and protecting the health of their children and others around them.

Current Treatment Options

When a child is diagnosed with mumps, prompt and effective management is essential to alleviate symptoms and prevent complications. Currently, there is no specific antiviral treatment for mumps; instead, care is primarily supportive. Parents should focus on ensuring that their child gets plenty of rest, stays hydrated, and receives over-the-counter pain relievers such as acetaminophen or ibuprofen to reduce fever and relieve discomfort. It is critical to monitor the child's symptoms and consult a healthcare provider if they worsen or if there are signs of complications.

In addition to symptomatic treatment, parents should be aware of the importance of isolation during the contagious period of mumps, which typically lasts from a few days before the onset of symptoms until five days after the swelling of the salivary glands begins. This measure is crucial not only for the well-being of the infected child but also for the wider community, as mumps is highly contagious. Keeping children home from school or daycare during this period can help prevent further spread of the virus.

For children with underlying health conditions or those who are immunocompromised, the management of mumps may require more careful consideration. Special attention should be paid to potential complications, such as orchitis in post-pubertal males or oophoritis in females, as these can lead to long-term issues like infertility. In these cases, healthcare providers might recommend additional monitoring and specialized care to address any complications that arise.

In the event of a mumps outbreak, public health officials may implement specific strategies to control the spread of the virus. This can include increasing vaccination efforts, especially in communities with low immunization rates. Parents should be proactive in understanding their child's vaccination status and the importance of the measles, mumps, and rubella (MMR) vaccine, as it is the most effective method of preventing mumps and its complications.

Lastly, it is vital for parents to stay informed about the latest advancements in mumps diagnosis and treatment. Ongoing research into viral infections and vaccines may yield new insights and improved approaches to managing mumps in the future. By keeping abreast of credible medical information and actively engaging in discussions with healthcare providers, parents can better navigate the complexities of mumps treatment and contribute to their child's health and safety.

Future Directions in Mumps Research

As researchers continue to unravel the complexities of mumps, future directions in mumps research are likely to focus on enhancing vaccination strategies and improving public health policies. One significant area of interest is the development of next-generation vaccines that could offer broader protection and longer-lasting immunity. Current vaccines have proven effective, but there is a need for formulations that can better address emerging strains and variations of the virus. Additionally, ongoing studies aim to understand the immune response triggered by existing vaccines, which could lead to improvements in dosage and administration schedules.

Another critical avenue for research involves understanding the long-term effects of mumps infections, particularly in immunocompromised populations. These individuals may experience more severe complications from mumps, and current knowledge about their specific risks and outcomes remains limited. Future studies will aim to provide clearer insights into how mumps exacerbates underlying health issues in these populations, which can inform tailored prevention strategies and treatment protocols.

Mumps outbreaks can occur in various settings, and research into outbreak response strategies is increasingly vital. By examining past outbreaks, especially in communities with low vaccination rates, researchers can identify effective measures for rapid response and containment. This includes developing guidelines that public health officials can utilize in real-time to mitigate the spread of mumps and protect vulnerable populations. Such insights could also enhance public awareness campaigns, emphasizing the importance of vaccinations and timely reporting of suspected cases.

Mumps transmission prevention methods are another key focus area. Investigating the role of social behaviors, travel patterns, and community dynamics in the spread of mumps can yield valuable information for enhancing prevention strategies. Understanding how mumps is transmitted in different environments, including schools and public gatherings, will enable health officials to implement targeted interventions. Furthermore, research on the impact of international travel on mumps outbreaks will be crucial, especially as global mobility increases.

Finally, addressing myths and misinformation surrounding mumps and its vaccination is essential for future research initiatives. Studies aimed at understanding the origins and spread of vaccine hesitancy will be critical in developing effective communication strategies. By identifying common misconceptions and the psychological factors that contribute to them, researchers can collaborate with public health organizations to create educational materials that resonate with parents. This effort is vital to ensuring that accurate information about mumps and vaccination reaches all communities, thereby fostering informed decision-making and promoting public health.

Chapter 9: Mumps and Public Health Policy

Role of Government in Vaccination Programs

The role of government in vaccination programs is critical, particularly in the context of mumps prevention. Governments are responsible for establishing policies that promote public health and ensure widespread vaccination coverage. This responsibility includes developing comprehensive vaccination schedules, funding immunization initiatives, and collaborating with healthcare providers to facilitate access to vaccines. By prioritizing mumps vaccination, governments can mitigate the risks associated with outbreaks, protect vulnerable populations, and ultimately reduce the incidence of mumps-related complications.

In addition to policy formulation, governments play a significant role in public education regarding the importance of vaccination. Mumps vaccination awareness campaigns are essential in dispelling myths and misinformation surrounding vaccines. By providing accurate information through various channels, such as social media, community outreach programs, and educational materials, governments can help parents understand the benefits of vaccination and the potential risks of not vaccinating their children. Such efforts are vital in fostering trust in vaccination programs and encouraging higher vaccination rates.

Moreover, governments must respond swiftly to mumps outbreaks to control transmission and protect public health. This involves coordinating with health departments, healthcare providers, and community organizations to implement outbreak response strategies. These strategies may include targeted vaccination campaigns in affected areas, contact tracing, and public health advisories. By taking decisive action during an outbreak, governments can reduce the spread of mumps and prevent further complications, particularly among immunocompromised populations who are at greater risk.

Historically, the impact of government-led vaccination initiatives has been significant in reducing the prevalence of mumps and other vaccine-preventable diseases. Vaccination programs have led to a dramatic decline in mumps cases since the introduction of the measles, mumps, and rubella (MMR) vaccine. Governments have learned from past epidemics, using data and historical trends to guide their public health policies. This knowledge informs proactive measures to prevent future outbreaks and protect public health, particularly as global travel increases and the risk of mumps transmission across borders becomes more pronounced.

Finally, the government's involvement in mumps vaccination extends to research and innovation in diagnosis and treatment advancements. By funding scientific research, governments can support the development of improved vaccines and therapeutic options for mumps. This investment in public health not only enhances the response to current challenges but also prepares health systems for future threats. By reinforcing the importance of vaccination and ensuring robust public health policies, governments can help secure a healthier future for children and communities, ultimately reducing the burden of mumps and its associated complications.

Policies for Outbreak Management

Effective outbreak management policies are essential for controlling the spread of mumps and protecting public health. These policies are designed to establish clear protocols for identifying, reporting, and responding to cases of mumps, particularly during periods of heightened transmission. Parents play a crucial role in this process by ensuring their children are vaccinated and maintaining awareness of local health advisories. Vaccination remains the first line of defense, as the MMR (measles, mumps, rubella) vaccine has proven highly effective in preventing mumps outbreaks.

In the event of a mumps outbreak, public health officials implement a series of measures aimed at controlling transmission. This includes immediate identification of cases through symptom recognition and laboratory confirmation. Parents should be vigilant about symptoms such as fever, swollen salivary glands, and aching jaws. Once cases are confirmed, contact tracing becomes vital. Public health authorities will identify individuals who have been in close contact with an infected person, ensuring they receive appropriate guidance regarding vaccination status and monitoring for symptoms.

Isolation of infected individuals is a key policy component during an outbreak. Infected persons are advised to stay home and avoid contact with others, particularly those who are unvaccinated or immunocompromised. This isolation period typically lasts until five days after the onset of symptoms. Schools and childcare facilities may also enact policies to prevent further spread, such as temporary closures, increased sanitation measures, and educational outreach to inform parents about the importance of vaccination and symptoms to watch for.

Communication is another critical aspect of outbreak management. Public health agencies often utilize multiple channels, including social media, community meetings, and local news outlets, to disseminate important information swiftly. Parents should remain informed through these updates to ensure they understand the current situation and the best practices for keeping their families safe. Additionally, addressing myths and misinformation about mumps and the MMR vaccine is essential to foster a well-informed community that supports vaccination efforts.

Finally, robust policies for managing mumps outbreaks must include a focus on vulnerable populations. Immunocompromised individuals are at a higher risk for severe complications from mumps and require extra precautions during an outbreak. Health authorities may recommend additional vaccinations or preventive measures for these groups. By fostering an understanding of these policies, parents can contribute to community resilience against mumps outbreaks, ensuring their children, and others, remain protected in the face of this preventable disease.

The Importance of Public Awareness Campaigns

Public awareness campaigns play a crucial role in educating parents about the importance of mumps vaccination and prevention strategies. These campaigns aim to disseminate accurate information regarding the risks associated with mumps, the effectiveness of vaccines, and the potential complications arising from the disease. Mumps, a viral infection that can lead to serious health issues, has seen a resurgence in some regions due to declining vaccination rates. By fostering public awareness, these initiatives help in dispelling myths and misinformation surrounding the disease and encourage parents to make informed choices for their children's health.

One of the primary objectives of public awareness campaigns is to highlight the historical impact of mumps epidemics. Throughout history, mumps has caused significant morbidity and has been linked to severe complications, such as orchitis, meningitis, and hearing loss. By sharing historical data and personal stories, these campaigns underscore the importance of vaccination in preventing outbreaks and protecting community health. Parents are more likely to understand the significance of vaccination when they are aware of the consequences that previous generations faced due to mumps.

In addition to addressing historical perspectives, effective public awareness campaigns focus on the current state of mumps outbreaks and response strategies. By informing parents about recent outbreaks and the communities affected, these campaigns provide a sense of urgency and relevance. Parents need to be aware of how mumps spreads, particularly in settings with high transmission potential, such as schools and daycare centers. Understanding the dynamics of mumps transmission can empower parents to take proactive measures in preventing infection, including ensuring their children are up to date on vaccinations.

Another vital aspect of public awareness campaigns is their focus on the specific challenges faced by immunocompromised populations. Children with weakened immune systems may not respond as well to vaccines, making them more susceptible to mumps and its complications. Campaigns that address this issue help parents recognize the importance of herd immunity and how widespread vaccination can protect vulnerable members of the community. By highlighting the interconnectedness of individual and community health, these initiatives encourage parents to view vaccination as a collective responsibility.

Finally, public awareness campaigns also play a significant role in educating parents about the advancements in mumps diagnosis and treatment. As medical science progresses, new methods for diagnosing and managing mumps are being developed, which can improve outcomes for those affected. By informing parents about these advancements and debunking myths related to mumps treatment, these campaigns contribute to a more informed public. Ultimately, when parents are equipped with reliable information, they are better positioned to advocate for their children's health and contribute to the broader public health efforts aimed at controlling mumps and other vaccine-preventable diseases.

Chapter 10: Myths and Misinformation about Mumps

Common Myths Surrounding Mumps

Common myths surround mumps, often leading to confusion and misunderstanding among parents regarding the disease and its implications for their children. One prevalent myth is that mumps is no longer a threat due to the widespread use of the measles, mumps, and rubella (MMR) vaccine. While vaccination has significantly reduced the incidence of mumps in many regions, outbreaks can still occur, particularly in communities with low vaccination rates. It is crucial for parents to recognize that mumps can still pose a risk, especially in settings where unvaccinated individuals gather, such as schools and camps.

Another common misconception is that mumps only affects children. In reality, mumps can infect individuals of any age, including adolescents and adults. The complications associated with mumps, such as orchitis in males and oophoritis in females, can lead to long-term health issues, including fertility problems. Parents should be aware that even if their children have received the MMR vaccine, it is still possible to contract mumps, albeit typically in a milder form. Understanding this can help parents make informed decisions about their family's vaccination and health strategies.

Many parents also believe that mumps is merely a mild illness, one that does not require serious concern. This belief can be misleading, as mumps can lead to severe complications, including meningitis and encephalitis, which can have lasting effects on health. Moreover, mumps can be particularly dangerous for immunocompromised individuals, who may experience more severe symptoms and complications. Educating parents about these potential risks can encourage them to take preventive measures seriously and prioritize vaccination as a means of protecting not only their children but also vulnerable populations.

A further myth persists that natural infection with mumps provides better immunity than vaccination. However, this notion is flawed. The MMR vaccine is designed to provide effective immunity without the risks associated with contracting the disease, such as complications and spread to others. Vaccination not only protects the individual but also contributes to herd immunity, reducing the likelihood of outbreaks. Parents should understand that vaccination remains the safest and most effective method of preventing mumps and its associated risks.

Lastly, misinformation often circulates regarding the safety and necessity of the MMR vaccine. Some parents may be concerned about alleged links between vaccines and various health issues, despite extensive research demonstrating the safety of vaccines. It is essential for parents to rely on credible sources of information, such as healthcare professionals and public health organizations, to dispel myths and make informed decisions about vaccinations. By arming themselves with accurate information, parents can protect their children from mumps and contribute to the overall health of their communities.

The Impact of Misinformation

The impact of misinformation surrounding mumps and vaccinations can have far-reaching consequences for public health. In recent years, the availability of information has increased dramatically, but much of it is inaccurate or misleading. Parents seeking to educate themselves about mumps, its risks, and the importance of vaccination often encounter conflicting narratives. This confusion can lead to hesitancy in vaccination, which is critical in preventing outbreaks and protecting vulnerable populations. Understanding how misinformation spreads and influences parental decisions is essential for fostering a more informed community regarding mumps prevention.

One of the most significant consequences of misinformation is the resurgence of diseases that were previously under control. Mumps, for instance, was largely eliminated in many regions due to effective vaccination campaigns. However, when parents choose not to vaccinate their children based on false claims about vaccine safety, herd immunity diminishes, allowing the virus to circulate. This situation not only places unvaccinated children at risk but also endangers those who are unable to be vaccinated due to medical reasons. The implications of this misinformation extend beyond individual family decisions; they can lead to widespread public health threats that challenge healthcare systems.

Misinformation can also exacerbate the complications associated with mumps. Parents may underestimate the severity of mumps, believing it to be a mild illness. However, mumps can lead to serious complications such as orchitis, meningitis, and hearing loss. When parents are misled into thinking that the risks of vaccination outweigh the risks of the disease, they may inadvertently endanger their children's health. Educating parents about the potential long-term effects of mumps and the protective benefits of vaccination is crucial in countering this misinformation and ensuring informed decision-making.

In the realm of international travel, misinformation can pose additional challenges. Parents planning to travel with their children may not be aware of the mumps vaccination requirements in different countries or the increased risk of exposure in certain areas. This lack of awareness can lead to unvaccinated children being placed at risk in environments where mumps is more prevalent. Public health policies often reflect the need for vaccination to mitigate these risks, but when parents are influenced by myths, the effectiveness of these policies can be undermined. Thus, accurate information is paramount for safe international travel and the prevention of mumps outbreaks.

Combating misinformation requires a multifaceted approach, including the dissemination of accurate information through trusted sources, community engagement, and open dialogue between healthcare providers and parents. Public health campaigns must focus on clarifying misconceptions about mumps and vaccinations, emphasizing the scientific evidence supporting vaccination, and highlighting the dangers of misinformation. By empowering parents with knowledge and fostering a community that values accurate information, we can work towards reducing the impact of misinformation and improving the overall health of our communities.

Strategies for Educating Others

Educating others about mumps and its prevention is crucial for fostering a community that values public health. As a parent, sharing accurate information with friends, family, and your local community can significantly influence attitudes toward mumps vaccination. Begin by familiarizing yourself with the historical impact of mumps epidemics, which can help illustrate the importance of vaccination. Highlighting past outbreaks can serve as a stark reminder of the consequences of low vaccination rates. Use concrete examples from history that demonstrate how mumps has affected populations, particularly in immunocompromised groups, to help others appreciate the seriousness of the disease.

When discussing mumps vaccination awareness, it is essential to provide clear, evidence-based information. Parents may have concerns or misconceptions about vaccines, often fueled by myths and misinformation. Equip yourself with facts from reputable sources such as the Centers for Disease Control and Prevention (CDC) and the World Health Organization (WHO). Clarifying the benefits of the MMR (measles, mumps, rubella) vaccine, its safety profile, and the potential complications of mumps, including orchitis and meningitis, can help alleviate fears and encourage informed decision-making. Personal stories or testimonials from parents who have witnessed the impacts of mumps can also be powerful tools in advocacy.

Mumps outbreak response strategies are another critical area where education can make a difference. Parents should be aware of what steps to take in the event of an outbreak and how to identify symptoms early. Educating others about the signs of mumps, such as swollen salivary glands and fever, can lead to quicker responses and better outcomes. Encourage discussions about how to maintain communication with local health officials and schools to stay informed about vaccination rates and potential outbreaks. Emphasizing the role of collective responsibility in preventing outbreaks can motivate parents to prioritize vaccination for their children.

In addition to individual actions, educating others about mumps transmission prevention methods is vital. Discuss the importance of good hygiene practices such as frequent handwashing, avoiding close contact with infected individuals, and the significance of vaccination as the primary defense against mumps. Providing practical tips for travel, especially international travel where mumps can be more prevalent, can further empower parents to protect their families. Encourage open conversations about vaccination status before travel and the necessity of ensuring all family members are up to date with their vaccinations.

Lastly, fostering a dialogue about mumps and public health policy can engage parents in broader discussions about health initiatives in their communities. Encourage them to advocate for policies that promote vaccination and address misinformation. Joining local health committees or attending community health meetings can provide opportunities for parents to influence public health decisions. Creating a supportive network where parents can share resources, ask questions, and discuss their concerns about mumps can help build a stronger community committed to health education and prevention efforts. By working together, parents can play a significant role in reducing the incidence of mumps and ensuring a healthier future for their children.

www.ingramcontent.com/pod-product-compliance
Lightning Source LLC
Chambersburg PA
CBHW061529250726
48657CB00005B/2159